MOMMA IS CONFUSED AND SO AM I

Knowing the Difference between Dementia and Alzheimer's Disease

CAROL L. HOWELL

ISBN- 9798692002822

TABLE OF CONTENTS

*That act of following
was a learning process
for the disciples. They
were not thrown into
the waters and advised
they needed to swim.*

*Jesus was there to
guide them.*

*We need that same
instruction so we can
be prepared for the
challenges of life with
dementia.*

IT BEGINS...

It was August of 2006 when my world changed, and the calm sea of my life started to experience some turbulence. The winds of confusion and forgetfulness blew in while waves of panic and fear pounded the shores. My beloved Momma had received a diagnosis of Alzheimer's type dementia.

Vera Jean Holder is my Momma, and her life story is why I write. Praying and hoping Momma's experience with Alzheimer's will result in an easier journey of dementia for other people, I work daily to help educate others.

I received the news of Momma's diagnosis over the phone. I still remember that day, and I often wish I could have a "heart-to-heart" with the doctor who decided it was appropriate to make such a life-changing announcement in such a cold and uncaring fashion. "Mrs. Howell, your mother has dementia." Point blank. To the point. No cushions to catch me when I fell.

"Are you telling me my mother might get dementia," I asked.

"No, ma'am. She has dementia. I will call her in some medicine. If you need anything, let me know."

End of story. It was as if he said, "I've done my part, goodbye."

After recovering from the shock, although I am not quite sure that ever happens, I began to research and learn. I found tidbits of information that made me hopeful, and I found tidbits of information that scared the life out of me. Throughout the process, though, I began to understand one consistent theme. "People need people."

We need each other to navigate life. All of it. When the bad times hit, and they certainly will, having a strong support team makes the journey across the rough seas more manageable. I am a woman of faith. My perspective of life is not influenced by my faith. Rather, faith is the basis, foundation, guide and process by which I try to lead every minute of the day. This journey of dementia—whether I liked it or not—with or without my invitation, was going to be faced with that same faith.

I recall the story of Jesus walking on the waters of the Sea of Galilee in Matthew 4:18-20:

> While walking by the Sea of Galilee, he saw two brothers, Simon (who is called Peter) and Andrew his brother, casting a net into the sea, for they were fishermen. And he said to them, 'Follow me, and I will make you fishers of men.' Immediately they left their nets and followed him.

Simon and Andrew were simply told to follow Jesus. They were not told what the journey would consist of or where the journey would lead. Just follow. They were told the most important part, though. This following would make them "fishers of men." That is what we are all called to be … "fishers of men." The men and women I am called to fish for are those that have dementia and their caregivers. You, as a caregiver, have been called to follow God as you "fish" for your loved one who is no longer able to fish for themselves.

They need to know of God's love, His hope, and His hand throughout their journey. This love and hope begins with a relationship with Christ, and it leads to a better understanding of dementia and the diseases that cause it. After all, Jesus told His disciples, "Follow me." That act of following was a learning process for the disciples. They were not thrown into the waters and advised they needed to swim. Jesus was there to guide them, instruct them, teach them, and love on them. As caregivers, we need that same instruction so we can be prepared for the challenges of life with dementia.

Let's begin our fishing expedition together. We will start with the difference between Dementia and Alzheimer's.

Dementia is caused by something, and that something needs to be explored. Knowing the type of dementia can direct the physician to proper medications.

"IT'S ONLY DEMENTIA"

I receive several phone calls a week from caregivers who are seeking help, information, and hope. I always ask what type dementia their loved one has been diagnosed with. It is not uncommon to hear, "It's just old age dementia." Old age and dementia do not have to go hand-in-hand.

Do you know anyone who is 70 or beyond that does not have dementia? Of course you do. That should be a clue that dementia has more to it than just age. On the flip side of that coin, do you know a young person, someone in their 50s, who has dementia? I hope you don't, but I know several folks who were struck with dementia early in their life.

If dementia is not an "old age condition," then what is it? Simply put, *dementia is the inability to think clearly.* I love to stop there in my explanation and see the reaction I receive from folks after making that statement. Most all the folks will have a blank stare and look of fright on their face. I can just see them thinking, "Oh no. I've got it!"

Statistically, many of those folks are correct. By the time we reach the age of 65, ten percent of us will have Alzheimer's-type dementia. By the time we reach the age of 85, fifty percent of us will have been diagnosed with this fatal disease.

Alzheimer's is the 6th leading cause of death in America, and it is the only disease for which there is no cure *and* no means to slow its progression. When I speak to groups, it startles me to think that half the group will one day have Alzheimer's. Further, the disease is busy destroying the brain many years before any symptom appears.

So, you think you know no one with Alzheimer's? Think again. These folks are all around you, and they may not yet know. We all need to learn about dementia and be prepared. Another statistic states that as of this writing (2016), one in five families know and/or care for someone with dementia. By the year 2023, that statistic is expected to read "one in two families know and/or care for someone with dementia." That is shocking. That is why I write, teach, lecture, and coach about dementia.

Now, let us add to the definition, "the inability to think clearly" the phrase "that affects the activities of daily living." In the medical community, the activities of daily living are described as bathing, eating, ambulating, dressing, and toileting. To help you remember this, I recommend the following acronym:
B E A D (like in a necklace) with a **T** on the end.

- **B–bathing–**Failure to bath regularly or inability to recall the processes involved in bathing become apparent.

- **E–eating–**Forgetting to eat or no longer recognizing food causes the individual to cease eating.
- **A–ambulating–**Walking turns to shuffling or "skiing," and falls become more likely.
- **D–dressing–**The inability to choose seasonally appropriate or occasion appropriate clothing becomes an issue. It is not uncommon to see an individual wear dirty clothing or multiple layers of clothing.
- **T–toileting–**Bowel and bladder incontinence becomes a problem. Individuals have difficulty remembering where the bathroom is located and how to recognize their need to void.

When at least two of these areas are affected or altered by the inability to think clearly, doctors will likely diagnose dementia. (I recommend using the SYMPTOMS CALENDAR at the end of this book to track changes in behavior. Use the calendar to clearly explain these changes to your physician.)

This dementia is *caused* by an outside source. Dementia, in and of itself, is not a disease. It is a manifestation of a disease, disorder or imbalance. Therefore, knowing the reason for the dementia becomes essential.

My clients often have no idea what the cause of their loved one's dementia might be. They will say, "It is just regular Alzheimer's," or, "It's just dementia – nothing special about it." Of course, this is inaccurate. Dementia is caused by something, and that something needs to be explored. Knowing the type of dementia can direct the physician to proper medications. Assuming an individual has Alzheimer's, when they have Parkinson's, can lead to improper medication management.

There are over 200 different causes of dementia. We will look at a few of the most common.

*Remember, if one day
granny seems fine, and
the next day she is
confused or agitated,
she needs immediate
medical attention.*

REVERSIBLE DEMENTIAS

Reversible dementias are, by definition, not permanent and may go away after the underlying conditions are treated. The following is a list of common medical issues that can cause reversible dementias. Questions are included not to diagnose your loved one but to help you become more aware of symptoms that might present in these cases. If you suspect that your loved one has any of these conditions, contact your physician right away.

Urinary Tract Infection

If a person seemed fine one day, and they become confused and/or agitated the next day, the doctor will most likely order a urinalysis to look for a urinary tract infection. This is especially true with senior citizens. A urinary tract infection can cause a range of emotional and behavioral changes in seniors. They may become weepy, sad, angry, aggressive, forgetful, confused, or all of the above. I have seen senior citizens become so agitated they tried to harm themselves and others because of the urinary tract infection they were experiencing. It is important to investigate this possibility because it is treatable. The proper course of antibiotics will clear up the infection, and the symptoms will often go away.

If an individual has already been diagnosed with dementia from another source, and they experience a sudden change in their behavior, ask for a urinalysis then, also. The symptoms of any type dementia can be amplified because of an infection anywhere in the body, but a urinary tract infection is very often the culprit.

An excellent way to prevent urinary tract infections is to ensure proper hydration. In addition, dehydration can cause dementia to worsen.

???

1. Does your loved one experience pain while urinating?

2. Does your loved one have a fever? (But note that some drugs for the elderly, like those for rheumatoid arthritis, may inhibit fevers.)

Tumors

Scriptures tell us we are "fearfully and wonderfully made; your works are wonderful, I know that full well" (Isaiah 139:14). I think of that scripture each time I am reminded of the dementia that can result from a tumor anywhere in the body. Sudden onset dementia can occur when a tumor grows within the body. Once the tumor is removed, the dementia will usually end. I am amazed at this particular process God has put into place to warn us that something is wrong with our bodies. Isn't God great?

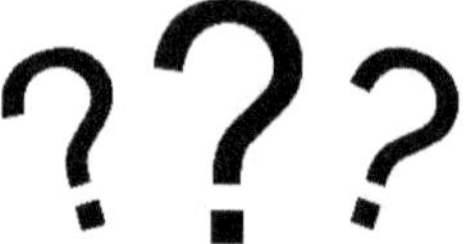

1. Is your loved one experiencing headaches that are different than headaches they have experienced previously?

2. Does your loved one have unexplained nausea, vomiting, swelling or a newly formed lump?

3. Does your loved one have a worsening condition—such as weight loss, difficulty breathing, or general pain—for which there is no explanation?

Vitamin B Deficiency

My mother-in-law was anemic and had a very low vitamin B level. The doctors tried to raise her level, but the success was minimal. Even so, her levels remained outside the normal range. As a result, she had dementia. She received vitamin B injections every-other-week, and her dementia improved for a few days. However, when it was time for an injection, her dementia symptoms increased.

If the vitamin B deficiency is discovered early and before the levels have plummeted too low, the process for raising the levels is more successful, and the dementia usually goes away.

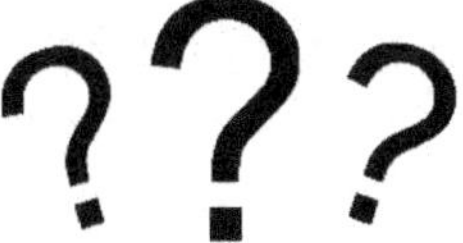

1. Is your loved one more tired or weak than before?

2. Does your loved one experience tingling, numbness, or muscle weakness, usually in the hands and feet?

Diabetes

My mother-in-law actually had two reasons to have dementia. She was diabetic. Anytime her sugar levels got out of control, her dementia was exacerbated. Once we got the sugar levels back into their normal range, she began to act more normally.

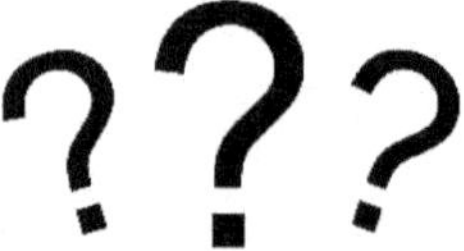

1. Is your loved one suddenly losing weight?

2. Is your loved one suddenly much hungrier or thirstier than normal?

3. Is your loved one going to the bathroom more frequently?

4. Does it take longer for your loved one's wounds (scratches, etc.) to heal?

Thyroidism

Thyroidism is caused by an imbalance in the thyroid hormone. This imbalance can be an excessive amount of the thyroid hormone (hyperthyroidism) or too little of the thyroid hormone (hypothyroidism). Thyroidism can lead to dementia and a host of other issues. Once the thyroid hormone balance is regulated, the dementia goes away.

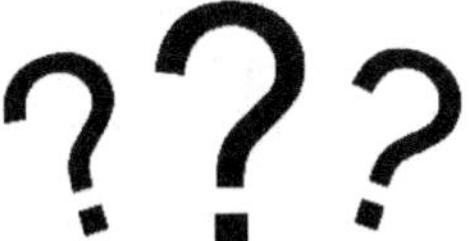

1. Is your loved one gaining or losing weight unexpectedly?

2. Is your loved one more tired than usual?

3. Does your loved one have excessive hair loss?

Adverse Effect of Legal Medications

Many of us have been around someone who took a new medication and started "acting strangely." My mother is the life of the party when she takes Nubain. She has very real hallucinations because of this medication. Once it leaves her system she is fine. This is an adverse effect from a prescribed medication that was taken properly.

Individuals who abuse prescribed medications will often experience dementia also. Once the drugs leave the system, the dementia usually goes away.

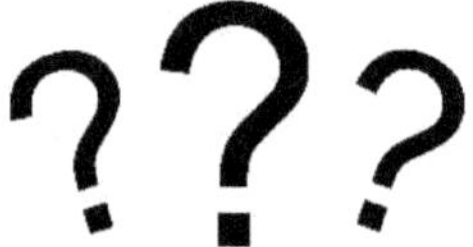

1. Check the labels of your loved one's medications. Is dementia or confusion listed as a side effect?

2. Does the dementia occur about the same time the medication begins to work (usually within an hour for many medications)?

Poisoning

Excess exposure to pesticides, chemicals, or heavy metals can lead to dementia that is reversible. Once these substances have been removed from the blood stream, the dementia goes away.

There is much discussion about exposure to aluminum. Controversy exists as to whether it is safe to use deodorant with aluminum, drink from aluminum cans, or eat food prepared in aluminum cookware. I tend to be conservative. If there is an easy way to reduce my chances of any type dementia, I follow that way. My deodorant is all natural, my sparkling water is in a bottle, and my cookware is stainless steel.

Speaking of water and aluminum, interesting research has been conducted by Dr. Christopher Exley. Dr. Exley is the Reader in Bioinorganic Chemistry at The Birchall Centre, Keele University in Staffordshire and Honorary Professor at the UHI Millennium Institute.

His research was geared toward discovering the impact of aluminum on the human body, specifically the brain. Our bodies need ZERO amounts of aluminum, yet autopsies of individuals who progressed through all the stages of Alzheimer's revealed substantial amounts of aluminum in their brains. There would seem to be a connection between aluminum and Alzheimer's.

To test this theory, a study was conducted with a test group and a control group. They were all administered cognitive tests to determine their levels of ability. The control group changed nothing in their daily routine. The test group drank one liter of silica rich water daily. After a period of time, cognitive tests were again administered to both groups.

The control group showed continuing decline in their cognitive ability. The test group showed an increase in their abilities! This is excellent news.
There are only three waters commercially available that contain naturally occurring silica. The most easily obtained is FIJI water. It can be found online and in most grocery stores. Another wonderful benefit from adding one liter of water a day is the reduced risk of dehydration and constipation.

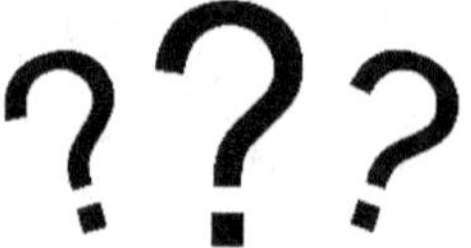

1. Is your loved one currently being exposed to chemicals for prolonged periods—for example, local construction projects or recent changes to the water supply.

2. Are there simple ways that you could decrease your loved one's exposures?

Illegal Drug and Alcohol Abuse

If you have ever watched television, you have witnessed dementia brought on by excessive alcohol consumption. This is true, also, for use of illegal drugs. Removing these substances from the blood stream will most often end the dementia. If the abuse has been on-going, permanent damage can occur.

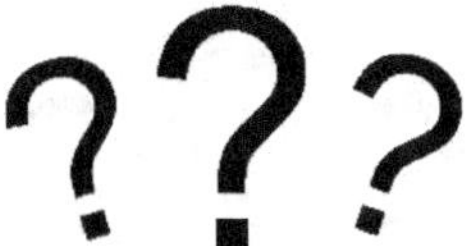

1. Has your loved one had a problem with drug or alcohol abuse in the past?

2. Have you discovered evidence of a substance abuse problem in your loved one's home?

Apoxia and Hypoxia

Apoxia is an insufficient amount of oxygen in the blood and tissues brought on by high altitudes.

Hypoxia is an insufficient amount of oxygen despite sufficient blood flow to the tissues. Both these conditions can bring about dementia. Once the situation is corrected, the dementia ends.

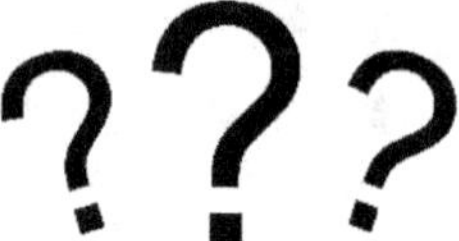

1. Have you noticed any changes in the skin coloring of your loved one? Changes might include a blue tinge around your loved one's lips or under their fingernails or their skin may become cherry red.

2. Have you noticed your loved one having difficulty breathing?

Remember, if one day granny seems fine, and the next day she is confused or agitated, she needs immediate medical attention. There is a very good chance she is in pain. Don't delay seeking help.

*Anything that is good
for the heart is also
good for the brain!*

IRREVERSIBLE DEMENTIAS OTHER THAN ALZHEIMER'S DISEASE

The dementias caused by many diseases are often termed "irreversible dementias." These include, but are not limited to, the following diseases.

Parkinson's Disease

One of the first symptoms of Parkinson's Disease is a change in the way a person moves, and it begins with a problem in certain nerve cells in the brain that produce dopamine. Dopamine is important because it communicates with the muscles to allow them to move and perform the way they are intended to move. When these nerve cells become damaged, and there is not enough dopamine, movement becomes a problem.

Parkinson's often manifests first with tremors of the extremities, balance issues, stiffened muscles, and slow movement. A later side effect would be dementia. Note, however, dementia is not the first symptom of Parkinson's Disease.

I personally have seen quite a few cases of Parkinson's Disease. Two very famous people with Parkinson's are Katharine Hepburn and Michael J. Fox.

Huntington's Disease

Huntington's Disease is a progressive brain disorder caused by a single defective gene on chromosome 4. It can develop as early as age 2 or as late in life as age 80, but it is most often noticed in midlife. The first symptoms of Huntington's disease are usually unsteady gait accompanied with uncontrolled movement of the arms, legs, face, and upper body. Dementia may follow at some point in the disease. Once again, dementia is not the first symptom of Huntington's Disease.

Lewy Body Disease

Lewy Body Disease is often misdiagnosed as Alzheimer's or Parkinson's Disease. Lewy Body Disease is caused by abnormal cells in the mid-brain region. Frederick Lewy discovered these cells, thus their name. The most common symptom is impairment in walking. This impairment results in a shuffling gait. It looks as if the person is skiing or skating. Muscle stiffness and a tendency to fall are common. Visual hallucinations often occur and are predominately focused on children, insets, and sexual activity. It is more common for someone with Lewy Body Disease Dementia to experience difficulty making good decisions. While dementia may be a result of Lewy Body Disease, the inability to remember is not the first symptom.

In my work, I have experienced many people with Lewy Body Disease. Each of these individuals was misdiagnosed originally, and their doctors later changed their diagnosis to Lewy Body Disease Dementia. One individual experienced sudden and uncontrolled tightening of his muscles. He would sit quietly and suddenly stand up and jerk uncontrollably. After the muscles relaxed, he was able to sit comfortably again for a few minutes.

Pick's Disease

Pick's Disease is often misdiagnosed as Alzheimer's. Dementia is common with Pick's Disease, but it is not the first symptom. Another name for Pick's Disease is "frontotemporal lobe dementia," as the frontal (that area behind your forehead) and temporal lobes (that area around your ears) of the brain are most affected by this disease. Because these areas are under attack, the first symptoms of Pick's Disease are usually a change in behavior and speech difficulty. The frontal lobe is responsible for distinguishing between appropriate and inappropriate behavior. When it becomes diseased, the result is a drastic change in behavior. Pick's Disease will present with this type of change in an individual's behavior before the presence of dementia is noted. Individuals will often become inappropriate, have outbursts of emotions, and not be in control of their words, actions or feelings.

Multi-Infarct Dementia (MID)/ Vascular Dementia

More commonly known as a stroke, the brain receives permanent damage that results in dementia. The stroke is usually caused by the presence of a clot in an artery in the brain. The region of the brain that strokes is the region that is damaged. High blood pressure puts a person at greater risk of having a stroke. Vascular Dementia is often listed as the 2nd most common type of dementia. Eating healthy and exercising are important in aiding the reduction of vascular diseases. Anything that is good for the heart is also good for the brain!

Normal Pressure Hydrocephalus (NPH)

Normal Pressure Hydrocephalus can result in a dementia that is reversible. I list it under "Irreversible Dementias" because it is most often misdiagnosed and mistreated, and this delay decreases the chances of a full return to cognitive function.

NPH is caused by a slow and gradual increase of the cerebrospinal fluid in the ventricles of the brain. The increase is not as dramatic as that of hydrocephalus. Thus, the term "normal pressure" comes into play. This increase in pressure, though, does begin to bring about problems. The most common symptoms of NPH are difficulties with the bladder and problems with walking.

When correctly diagnosed, NPH can be often be reversed by placing a shunt in the head to drain the excess cerebrospinal fluid. This process then reduces the pressure on the ventricles.

I have a client who was diagnosed with Alzheimer's. After meeting with him and his wife several times, I was not convinced his diagnosis was correct. Thus began the process of visiting many doctors and teaching hospitals. After about four months, this man was diagnosed with NPH. A shunt was installed on the right side of his forehead. This shunt drained the excess cerebrospinal fluid into his abdomen.

After returning to our coaching sessions, I was amazed and thrilled to observe the changes he experienced due to the proper diagnosis and treatment. He went from barely being able to lift his feet to walk, to walking normally. He went from having rigid uncontrolled muscles, to sitting still and relaxed. He could navigate his way through his home, the grocery store, and local restaurants without getting lost. His dementia decreased dramatically. It was a huge success story!

Subdural Hematoma

A subdural hematoma is bleeding between the brain and its protective outer layer. This usually occurs due to trauma to the head. This trauma may be referred to as a "closed head injury," and the hematoma may not be immediately detected. It is important to seek immediate medical attention after a head injury to rule out the presence of a subdural hematoma. However, the hematoma can result in dementia.

A closed-head injury is all too familiar to my family and me. My husband sustained such an injury in 1992. His injury resulted in loss of his memory for a four-year span of time. When he awoke from the accident that caused his injury, he did not recognize me, recall we were married, remember his daughter, had no idea what his job was, recall what type car he drove, recognize his own home, or many other activities we all take for granted.

After eighteen months, eight hours a day, of physical therapy and visual therapy, my husband was able to return to "normal" life. I put the word "normal" in quotes, as it is used cautiously in this story. He will never remember all the events that happened during that time frame. However, we are so blessed to have each other. I wouldn't trade him for anyone!

Down Syndrome

Down Syndrome is caused by a genetic disorder. A person is born with 47 chromosomes instead of 46. This syndrome is identified at birth. Dementia can result.

It is my pleasure to conduct Creative Music Experiences with several individuals who have Down Syndrome. These particular friends know how to enjoy life despite the disabilities they experience.

Creutzfeldt-Jakob Disease

More commonly known as Mad Cow Disease, it is also known as Bovine Spongiform Encephalopathy when present in cattle. The disease is transmitted to humans who have eaten food contaminated with the disease. Its presence in cattle usually occurs when the animals have been fed other cattle rather than grain. The human form is called Creutzfeldt-Jakob Disease.

While this disease is rare, I have a client whose mother died from this progressive and ravaging disease. My client was told the odds of her mother having Creutzfeldt-Jakob Disease was one in a million, yet it happened. What amazes me more is this same client met a neighbor who had a relative die of the same disease. One common link is both diagnosed individuals had traveled outside the country prior to their diagnoses.

Acquired Immune Deficiency Syndrome (AIDS)

Acquired Immune Deficiency Syndrome (AIDS) is caused by Human Immunodeficiency Virus (HIV). This virus attacks the immune system which makes the body more susceptible to many illnesses and life-threatening conditions. Dementia can be a symptom of AIDS, but it is not the first symptom.

There are many diseases that can cause dementia. Besides Alzheimer's, these are the most common. There are over 200 different reasons a person may have a reversible or irreversible dementia. If you count all those people, there are more people with Alzheimer's dementia than the total of all the other dementias. Let's look at Alzheimer's dementia in more detail.

It is disturbing to realize the processes that are taking place, but it is important to have a basic understanding.

This knowledge will lead to power. That power will lead to hope. Hope will lead to smiles. Don't we all need more smiles?

WHAT IS ALZHEIMER'S DISEASE?

Simply put, Alzheimer's Disease is a disease of the brain. The hallmark symptom of Alzheimer's is always memory loss. There is a good reason for that.

The first area of the brain to be affected by Alzheimer's is the hippocampus. The hippocampus is a dual lobe part of the brain (right side and left side), and it is located in its mid-region. Every new piece of information that enters the brain will first make a visit to the hippocampus. The healthy hippocampus will hold this information until such time as it moves that information to another place in the brain. This move takes place when an individual enters the dream stage of sleep. Deep sleep is important for our cognitive health. When information moves from the hippocampus to another part of the brain, it remains there and can be easily accessed when needed. Alzheimer's, however, makes it very difficult for information in the hippocampus to move to another part of the brain.

It is simple to remember this by thinking of the hippocampus as the "cardboard file box" for important information. Once that information becomes important enough to be retained, it is moved to a "steel file box" elsewhere in the brain where it will remain.

Alzheimer's Disease complicates the process. It attacks the hippocampus by destroying it from the inside out. It shrinks the hippocampus, and it causes a gap to form around the hippocampus. The new information entering the brain may try to land and stay on the hippocampus, but this information is lost because of the disease within the hippocampus. If that information periodically finds a place to land on the hippocampus, the gap that is around the hippocampus prevents the information from moving to a permanent site in the brain.

This would explain why you may tell your loved one they have an appointment tomorrow at two o'clock, and they will not remember that information just a few minutes later. The information tried to attach to the hippocampus, but Alzheimer's Disease prevented the hippocampus from being able to accept that information.

Many folks are often perplexed when their loved one cannot remember information just given them, but they can tell stories from 1952. Let me help you understand why this is true.

The new information, as we just learned, is trying to be stored inside the hippocampus. Because of Alzheimer's Disease, the hippocampus cannot retain the information. However, old stories and memories from much earlier in life moved from the hippocampus to a permanent storage site in the brain many years ago. These stories are accessible. The further back in time the stories reach, the more likely the individual will be to recall them.

As Alzheimer's destroys memories, the most recent memories are lost first. For example, memories of great grandchildren will be lost before memories of grandchildren. Memories of grandchildren will be lost before memories of children. The memories are lost in the reverse order in which they were gained.

It is safe to assume an individual will never forget their parents, grandparents, and any older sibling. These individuals existed before the individual was born, and these memories are stored in the far reaches of the brain. Because Alzheimer's tends to destroy the brain from the center out, the memories in the outer most regions of the brain are generally preserved. Now you might understand why a 90-year-old woman will say, "Please take me home to Momma." Her mind is pulling on the information that remains. That information is her momma.

As Alzheimer's Disease progresses, it eventually attacks the entire brain. It is disturbing to realize the processes that are taking place, but it is important to have a basic understanding. This knowledge will lead to power. That power will lead to hope. Hope will lead to smiles. Don't we all need more smiles?

Alzheimer's Disease is known for the plaque that develops on the brain. When we hear the word "plaque," we often think of the heart or teeth. Plaque can certainly accumulate in the heart and on teeth, and it can accumulate in the brain.

The healthy brain has over 100 billion neurons. Each of these neurons has protrusions called branches. It is estimated that the healthy brain has over 100 trillion branches. When neurons connect to each other through a small electrical charge, it is called a synapse. At this point, a release of chemicals occurs which is referred to as neurotransmitters. The neurotransmitters carry information to other neurons. Alzheimer's destroys this entire process through a substance known as beta-amyloid plaque composed of abnormal protein matter. Beta-Amyloid plaque comes between the neurons and prevents the information from being moved around the brain.

In addition to beta-amyloid plaque, there is a substance known as tau (which rhymes with cow). Tau gets inside the neurons and causes damage from the inside out. The inside of a neuron has a nice straight path. When tau invades, these paths become tangled, fall apart, and disintegrate. As a result, nutrients cannot travel within the cells. This causes the death of the cell.

As Alzheimer's Disease progresses, the brain matter itself begins to disintegrate. Brain matter actually leaves the body. By the time an individual is in the last stage of Alzheimer's, the brain has decreased to one-third of its original size. There are holes throughout the brain tissue that remains. The neurons are diseased from the inside out, the brain tissues turn an unhealthy color, and beta-amyloid plaque is hindering communication from one neuron to another. This is disturbing to imagine. However, it is important to realize that all the knowledge, memory, and abilities contained within that brain matter also leave the body.

My interactions with Momma are more meaningful when I accept her as she is. I do not try to change her.

WHY BOTHER?

This understanding of Alzheimer's should help us become better caregivers. When we cease expecting the unobtainable, we release stress for ourselves and our loved ones. My interactions with Momma are more meaningful when I accept her as she is. I do not try to change her. Loving her and caring for her as she is, on any given day, make us both happier.

It is important to understand how your loved one views their dementia. With few exceptions, the individual with dementia knew something was wrong with their ability to remember long before you, the caregiver, noticed a problem. They realized a sense of confusion and forgetfulness that led to stress and even irritability. While trying to cover these issues (many people with dementia are excellent actors), they were able to hide or mask their symptoms. The symptoms became more difficult to hide as the disease progressed.

Recognizing changes in our loved ones is important throughout the aging process. Whether changes are a result of dementia or not, the changes need to be identified and investigated.

*Cross interaction
between individuals
brings about a sense of
peace, and a continued
sense of home. Home is
a beautiful word!*

IS IT TIME FOR ASSISTED LIVING CARE?

Early detection of the reason for dementia is key to the best possible outcome. While the outcome of Alzheimer's type dementia is never good, it can be improved with early detection. Don't delay in taking the steps necessary to determine the cause of a change in behavior. Don't settle for the diagnosis of "Dementia." Investigate until a reason for the dementia is made clear. If the reason is a reversible dementia, you can celebrate and correct the problem. If the reason is an irreversible dementia, you can make the proper decisions to bring the best quality of life to your loved one.

Speaking of the best quality of life for your loved one, realize that moving to an assisted living or group home is often one of the best decisions we can make for our loved one with dementia. My Momma blessed us greatly when she made the decision to move to an assisted living community. Momma and I visited the community because we were nosey! We just wanted to see what was being built. To top it off, we registered for a $100 gift card and won it!

During the tour, I noticed Momma was very interested. She asked many questions, and it all made me a little nervous. Momma was still working at the time. She spent her career in sales, and she was an amazing sales lady. Everywhere she worked, she gained the title "Top Sales Lady." She could convince you to purchase furniture—and later jewelry—that you didn't even know you wanted! This meant big commission checks that Momma loved to spend on her children. Life was good.

I realized Momma was experiencing cognitive issues, but I very much wanted to pretend they were "not that bad." In fact, Momma realized how difficult her working world had become due to her inability to think clearly. She received complaints from supervisors about invoices completed inaccurately, wrong directions for deliveries, and other such problems. Momma was quick to correct her problems, but the number of instances began to grow.

While touring the new assisted living, Momma realized she needed to make the decision to move. She looked at me and said, "Carol, I want to move here. You figure out how to pay for it!" I was shocked Momma wanted to move. I was also very perplexed as to how we could possibly afford the move.

Thankfully, Momma had purchased a long-term care insurance policy about five years prior to her decision to move. This policy was easily activated because Momma already had a medical diagnosis of Alzheimer's-type dementia. So, the move was made. Her long-term care insurance policy made the move very affordable. I am forever grateful she made that purchase those many years ago, and I will be purchasing a policy for myself when I turn 60. Maybe you should also!

Interestingly, Momma was still working every day when she moved to the assisted living, and she drove herself to work daily. This went on for about eighteen months, and one day Momma started having trouble with directions.

I recall that day very vividly. Momma called me very upset. She had left her assisted living to go to the family doctor for a routine checkup. She was lost. She could not remember which way to turn, could not get her thoughts together to determine where she was at that moment in time, and she was embarrassed, frustrated, and sad. I helped her through this situation, but my heart sank.

It was only a few days later Momma decided she should not drive any longer. Her car was sold, and I began the process of helping her get to work daily. She worked fewer days a week at that time, and those days decreased as the dementia progressed.

However, Momma's decision to move to an assisted living was key to her long-term health and wellbeing. Studies have proven that individuals with dementia live longer and have a better quality of life when they live in a group setting such as an assisted living facility. Many families find this hard to believe. I often have family members say, "I want to keep Momma home until we just can't care for her any longer." Hmm… let's think about that.

While you are keeping Momma home trying to care for her, you are also trying to work, maintain a family life, upkeep the house and yard, pay the bills, buy the groceries, clean the house, do the laundry, care for the children and grandchildren and on and on the list goes. How can all this be accomplished without outside assistance? It can't. Something will go lacking. Often times that lack will appear in the care and social stimulation the individual with dementia receives.

Social stimulation is key to our good health. This is true no matter our physical well-being. Time spent with friends, good conversation, activities that are engaging, music enjoyed, and food shared all bring about a feeling of happiness and good will. You experience this in your life as a healthy individual, and it becomes more important once dementia is part of the story.

Assisted living relieves you, the caregiver, of many responsibilities. A good assisted living will take care of both the physical and social needs of its residents. This allows you to visit your loved one and just be their daughter, son, grandchild, or spouse. You are no longer the caregiver. The peace that arises from this change in roles is amazing. You feel it, and your loved one does also.

IS IT TIME FOR ASSISTED LIVING CARE?

Even if you have many folks helping with the care of a loved one at home, the likelihood they will need group living at some point is high. Waiting until an individual has to move is not a good plan. Moving an individual while they can still participate in life, enjoy activities, make friends, and make their new apartment their home is key to a good future. Waiting until they must move often prohibits them from making the transition as easily as possible. Adjusting to and dealing with so many physical and cognitive issues make acclimating to the community more difficult.

If the decision to move to an assisted living has been made, be sure to choose a community that offers the levels of care you may need. Many communities are assisted living only. They do not offer a memory care community. If your loved one has moved because of a diagnosis of dementia, there is a strong possibility they will need memory care living during the last stages of their life. If the community you choose has memory care, the individual can transition from one part of the building to another part with great ease. If the community does not have memory care, a move to an entirely new community must take place. This move can be difficult for your loved one.

Why does your loved one care if they move from one building to another versus moving from one community to another? After all, they have dementia and will not remember. Good question.

Most communities will interact between their assisted living and memory care communities. Staff will visit between both communities, and the residents are often involved in activities in both communities. This cross interaction allows familiarity to exist. This brings about a sense of peace, and a continued sense of home. Home is a beautiful word!

*We are to love and care
for God's people. This
does not change in the
face of disease of any
kind.*

*However, we need to
have a community of
friends helping us make
life as beautiful as
possible.*

PULLING IT ALL TOGETHER

We spend our days making sure all our "p's and q's" are lined up. We want everyone to be happy, content, safe, well fed, well cared for, and most of all, loved. Making all this happen can be tiring. We are called to care for our family members. The Ten Commandments teach us to "Honour thy father and thy mother: that thy days may be long upon the land which the LORD thy God giveth thee." (Exodus 20:12). We are taught to care for the widows. "Support the widows who are in need" (I Timothy 5:3). We vowed to love our spouses "till death do us part." We are to love and care for God's people. This does not change in the face of disease of any kind.

However, we need to have a community of friends helping us make life as beautiful as possible. Don't travel the journey of dementia caregiving alone. Here is a less-than-comprehensive list of things you will need to be successful:

- You need help.
- You need support.
- You need dementia education.
- You need a helping hand.
- You need some who will allow you to cry on their shoulder.
- You need a quiet place to which you can escape and find solitude.

- You need to allow yourself to cry, scream and even yell at God—He doesn't mind if you yell at Him.
- You need to engage in stress reduction activities on a regular basis—exercise, yoga, meditation.
- You need good nutrition daily.
- You need to maintain regular visits to your physician.
- You need time to go to the nail and hair salon.
- You need time to shop—alone!
- You need other people.
- Most of all, you need a close relationship with The Lord Jesus as you seek His guidance, peace, direction, love, grace, mercy, and hope.

*No matter what lies
ahead in our journey of
dementia together, my
family and I are joining
hands with our Lord to
allow Him to lead
while we follow.*

IN CONCLUSION

Alzheimer's Disease is a scary and fatal disease. My grandmother died of it, and my mother has been diagnosed with it. I do not fight it! That comes as a surprise to most people. Instead, I am learning to live with it.

Matthew 28:20 says, "Teaching them to observe all things whatsoever I have commanded you: and, lo, I am with you always, *even* unto the end of the world. Amen." I take comfort in knowing God is with me. God is with my momma. No matter what lies ahead in our journey of dementia together, my family and I are joining hands with our Lord to allow Him to lead while we follow.

Thinking back to the story of Jesus telling His disciples to follow Him, I am uplifted to know He didn't leave them alone. He will not leave me. God's mercy and grace are mine. They are made fresh each day. Great is His faithfulness… even in the face of dementia.

SYMPTOMS CALENDAR

The following pages contain a daily calendar that you or your loved one's caregiver can use to chart your loved one's activities of daily living. Its purpose is to help you communicate your concerns with your loved one's physician more effectively by providing them with information they can readily use to understand the issues your loved one is experiencing.

The pages are divided into two sections.

The first section provides a page-per-day for you to take notes. Simply date the pages and describe any difficulties your loved one had with their daily activities of living. There is ample space to make more detailed notes.

The second section is a calendar with the month on a single page where you can tick off the problem areas your loved one experienced on any given day. This section will let your loved one's physician see, at a glance, how frequently these issues are occurring.

Day 1:

Date:

Bathing:

Eating:

Ambulating:

Dressing:

Toileting:

Day 2:

Date: ___________________________

Bathing:

____

Eating:

____

Ambulating:

____

Dressing:

____

Toileting:

____

Day 3:

Date:

Bathing:

Eating:

Ambulating:

Dressing:

Toileting:

Day 4:

Date: ________________________

Bathing:

____

Eating:

____

Ambulating:

____

Dressing:

____

Toileting:

____

Day 5:

Date:
____

Bathing:

____

Eating:

____

Ambulating:

____

Dressing:

____

Toileting:

____

Day 6:

Date: _______________________________

Bathing:

____

Eating:

____

Ambulating:

____

Dressing:

____

Toileting:

____

Day 7:

Date:

Bathing:

Eating:

Ambulating:

Dressing:

Toileting:

Day 8:

Date:

Bathing:

Eating:

Ambulating:

Dressing:

Toileting:

Day 9:

Date:

Bathing:

Eating:

Ambulating:

Dressing:

Toileting:

Day 10:

Date: _______________________________

Bathing:

____

Eating:

____

Ambulating:

____

Dressing:

____

Toileting:

____

Day 11:

Date:

Bathing:

Eating:

Ambulating:

Dressing:

Toileting:

Day 12:

Date:

Bathing:

Eating:

Ambulating:

Dressing:

Toileting:

Day 13:

Date:

Bathing:

Eating:

Ambulating:

Dressing:

Toileting:

Day 14:

Date: _______________________________

Bathing:

____

Eating:

____

Ambulating:

____

Dressing:

____

Toileting:

____

Day 15:

Date:

Bathing:

Eating:

Ambulating:

Dressing:

Toileting:

Day 16:

Date:
____

Bathing:

____

Eating:

____

Ambulating:

____

Dressing:

____

Toileting:

____

Day 17:

Date:
Bathing:

Eating:

Ambulating:

Dressing:

Toileting:

Day 18:

Date:

Bathing:

Eating:

Ambulating:

Dressing:

Toileting:

Day 19:

Date:

Bathing:

Eating:

Ambulating:

Dressing:

Toileting:

Day 20:

Date: _______________________________

Bathing:

____

Eating:

____

Ambulating:

____

Dressing:

____

Toileting:

____

Day 21:

Date:

Bathing:

Eating:

Ambulating:

Dressing:

Toileting:

Day 22:

Date:
____

Bathing:

____

Eating:

____

Ambulating:

____

Dressing:

____

Toileting:

____

Day 23:

Date:

Bathing:

Eating:

Ambulating:

Dressing:

Toileting:

Day 24:

Date: ___________________________

Bathing:

____

Eating:

____

Ambulating:

____

Dressing:

____

Toileting:

____

Day 25:

Date:
____

Bathing:

____

Eating:

____

Ambulating:

____

Dressing:

____

Toileting:

____

Day 26:

Date: ______________________

Bathing:

Eating:

Ambulating:

Dressing:

Toileting:

Day 27:

Date:

Bathing:

Eating:

Ambulating:

Dressing:

Toileting:

Day 28:

Date: _______________________

Bathing:

____

Eating:

____

Ambulating:

____

Dressing:

____

Toileting:

____

Day 29:

Date: ____________________________________

Bathing:

____

Eating:

____

Ambulating:

____

Dressing:

____

Toileting:

____

Day 30:

Date:

Bathing:

Eating:

Ambulating:

Dressing:

Toileting:

30 DAY OVERVIEW:

Highlight the problems experienced each day.

1	2	3	4	5	6	7
B E A D T	B E A D T	B E A D T	B E A D T	B E A D T	B E A D T	B E A D T
8	9	10	11	12	13	14
B E A D T	B E A D T	B E A D T	B E A D T	B E A D T	B E A D T	B E A D T
15	16	17	18	19	20	21
B E A D T	B E A D T	B E A D T	B E A D T	B E A D T	B E A D T	B E A D T
22	23	24	25	26	27	28
B E A D T	B E A D T	B E A D T	B E A D T	B E A D T	B E A D T	B E A D T
29	30					
B E A D T	B E A D T					

ABOUT THE AUTHOR

Carol Howell is the author of the #1 Amazon Best Seller *LET'S TALK DEMENTIA: A Caregiver's Guide.* It is available in paperback and e-reader formats through Amazon. You can check out Carol's website at www.seniorlifejourneys.com where you can download her podcast titled "LET'S TALK DEMENTIA" (also available on iTunes), view her video series, or purchase paperback copies of her books.

Carol Howell is Executive Director of Senior Life Journeys, a not for profit. She welcomes your questions through email. Contact her at carol@letstalkdementia.org.

If you are seeking an engaging and humorous speaker on the topic of dementia, write Carol for availability and pricing — carol@seniorlifejourneys.com.

Blessings and smiles!

MORE FROM CAROL HOWELL

Let's Talk Dementia

Carol Howell, Certified Dementia Practitioner and caregiver to her mother, helps to educate the reader on the various forms of dementia. She also provides hands-on tips that make life easier for the caregiver and better for the loved one with dementia. The book is scattered with "smiles" that brighten the day. The author reminds the readers of her motto—"Knowledge brings POWER. Power brings HOPE, and HOPE brings SMILES." You've just got to laugh!

If My Body Is a Temple, Why Am I Eating Doughnuts?

Have you tried to change your body and found it terribly difficult to accomplish? Have you looked in the mirror only to see an image with which you were not happy? That is exactly the way I have lived most of my life. This book tells you of the physical miracle I have experienced and the miracle of learning to love myself just like I am at any minute of any day. Then I learned God loves me even more! He loves me with all my cellulite, love handles, and belly. His love is not dependent upon my being a certain size or shape. You are about to begin a nine-week journey filled with personal stories and daily devotions. Along the way, you will discover the YOU that GOD made! So, put the doughnuts in the bottom of the trash can, empty the litter box on top of them, close the lid, and let's get down to work. I can't wait to see the NEW YOU!

REMINISCE AND WORSHIP

This full-color book is a 30-day devotional designed for the individual with dementia. The beautiful color pictures will bring to mind events from the past. The pictures are followed by scripture that relates to the picture and questions to ponder. The individual who can no longer read on their own will benefit by having a caregiver read the scriptures and aloud and interact with the individual using the questions following the scripture.